I0701938

ZERO-CARB DIET

FOR NOVICES

Enriched Recipes, Foods, Meal Plan & Procedures That Focuses On Guide To Low Carbohydrate, Weight Management And Healthy Living

DR. MATEO GABRIEL

Copyright © [Dr. Mateo Gabriel] [2003]. All rights reserved. You can't copy, distribute, or send any part of this book in any way, including by photocopying, recording, or other electronic or mechanical means, without the publisher's written permission first. The only times this is okay are for short quotes in reviews and other legal noncommercial uses.

DISCLAIMER

The information in this book is only meant to be used for general reading. In any way, the author and publisher do not promise or represent that the information in this work is full, correct, reliable, appropriate, or available. This includes any warranties that are expressed or implied. Because of this, you should only rely on this material at your own risk.

This book is not meant to replace professional help. If you have any questions about a subject, you should always get help from a qualified expert. The author and distributor of this book are not responsible for how the information in it is used or abused.

The author's thoughts and feelings are shown in this book. They do not necessarily represent the official policy or stance of any other person, group, employer, or business.

Any third-party material that you can get to through this book is not endorsed or backed by the author or publisher.

The information in this book is correct at the time it was published, after all possible checks. However, the author and distributor are not responsible for any loss, damage, or inconvenience that may be caused by mistakes or omissions.

TABLE OF CONTENTS

CHAPTER ONE

INTRODUCTION TO ZERO-CARB DIET

AN OUTLINE OF THE KETOGENIC DIET

The Carnivore Diet sometimes referred to as the Zero Carb Diet, is a dietary strategy that emphasizes the consumption of only animal products while limiting carbohydrate intake to almost nothing. Recent years have seen a rise in the popularity of this diet plan, with supporters citing several health advantages and successful weight reduction results.

Gaining knowledge of the foundational ideas, background, advantages, and debates around the Zero Carb Diet helps one comprehend the concept and consequences of the diet.

PRINCIPLES AND DEFINITION

The tight restriction of carbs, together with the elimination of all plant-based foods and an emphasis only on animal products, characterize the Zero Carb Diet. Proponents contend that this diet is consistent with human evolution, claiming that animal meat was the primary food source for early humans. To reach a state of ketosis, the main idea is to cut off all sources of carbohydrates, such as grains, fruits, vegetables, and even some dairy products. The body starts using fat for energy instead of carbs when it is in this metabolic state.

HISTORICAL CONTEXT

There is a link between the Zero Carb Diet and previous low-carb and ketogenic diets when one looks at its historical background. The early 20th-century work of doctors and scientists investigating the therapeutic advantages of carbohydrate restriction for diseases like epilepsy laid the groundwork for this strategy. The Zero Carb Diet differs from other low-carb diets in that it only emphasizes animal items;

other low-carb diets may occasionally incorporate plant-based foods.

The Zero Carb Diet's proponents list several possible advantages for this dietary strategy. When the body switches to burning fat for fuel, weight loss is a frequently observed consequence. Advocates also report higher energy levels, more mental clarity, and better control over specific medical illnesses like gastrointestinal problems and autoimmune disorders. It is important to remember that there is little scientific proof to back up these assertions, and it is unclear what the long-term consequences of adhering to such a rigid diet would be.

ADVANTAGES AND DEBATES

There is controversy about the zero-carb diet. Healthcare professionals and nutrition specialists frequently voice worries regarding the possible nutritional inadequacies linked to the avoidance of plant-based diets. Some who disagree contend that eating too little dietary fiber, vitamins, and phytonutrients from fruits and vegetables can be harmful to one's general health. The diet's sustainability and potential for negative impacts on cardiovascular health and cholesterol levels further raise concerns about its long-term feasibility.

The Zero Carb Diet is a distinct and contentious nutritional approach that is distinguished by its severe carbohydrate restriction and sole dependence on animal sources. Comprehending the definition, tenets, historical background, and related advantages and disputes is vital for those contemplating or assessing the consequences of embracing such a dietary plan.

CHAPTER TWO

THE SCIENCE OF CARBOHYDRATE ZERO

SUGARS AND CARBS

One of the three macronutrients—along with proteins and fats—carbohydrates are essential for giving the body energy. The atoms that make up these organic molecules are carbon, hydrogen, and oxygen, usually in the 1:2:1 ratio. Carbohydrates are primarily used by the body as a fast and effective source of energy for many physiological functions.

CARBS, SIMPLE VS. COMPLEX

Simple and complex carbs are the two basic categories into which carbohydrates can be generally divided. Simple carbohydrates are made up of one or two sugar units and are easily absorbed by the body, causing blood sugar levels to rise sharply.

Simple carbohydrates are frequently found in fruit sugars, honey, and refined sugars. Conversely, complex carbohydrates have a more intricate molecular structure since they are made up of several connected sugar units. Rich sources of complex carbs include vegetables, legumes, and whole grains.

Complex carbohydrates release energy more gradually because they take longer to break down.

INSULIN AND CARBOHYDRATES

The interaction between insulin and carbs is a vital component of metabolic processes. Upon ingestion, carbohydrates are converted to glucose, which is then released into the bloodstream. The pancreas secretes the hormone insulin in reaction to elevated blood sugar levels, which aids in the uptake of glucose by cells for storage or energy. Insulin is released in greater amounts to maintain glucose homeostasis when blood sugar rises more quickly, as is the case with simple carbohydrates.

Simple carbohydrate overconsumption over time can cause insulin resistance, a state in which cells lose their insulin sensitivity, which may aid in the onset of type 2 diabetes.

THE FUNCTION OF GLYCEROL IN THE BODY

The body uses carbohydrates as its main energy source, especially for critical organs like the muscles and brain. After being consumed, carbohydrates are transformed into glucose, which can either be used right away as fuel or stored as glycogen in the muscles and liver for later use.

This glycogen functions as an easily accessible energy source when fasting or engaging in greater physical activity occurs.

Furthermore, carbohydrates promote several metabolic processes, such as the creation of specific proteins and the control of blood sugar levels.

Advocates of low- or zero-carb diets contend that by reducing the amount of carbohydrates consumed, the body is compelled to use other fuel sources, such as ketones created during the breakdown of fat, a condition known as ketosis.

Even if some people might benefit from such dietary methods, it's important to take into account that everyone has a different metabolism and set of nutritional needs. It is essential to pay close attention to the kind and caliber of carbs ingested to preserve general health and well-being.

CHAPTER THREE

DIET ZERO CARB AND KETOSIS

A zero-carb diet, sometimes referred to as a ketogenic or low-carb diet, attempts to limit carbohydrates to the point that the body experiences a state called ketosis. When the body breaks down fat for energy in the absence of enough carbohydrates, it produces ketone bodies, which are high in the circulation and indicative of a metabolic state known as ketosis. This procedure is a cornerstone of the zero-carb diet theory since its proponents think it can have several health advantages.

THE KETOSIS PROCESS

The body uses its stored fat as its main energy source when the amount of carbohydrates it consumes is restricted. Ketones are water-soluble chemicals that the liver converts fats into so that cells can use them as fuel. When the body doesn't get enough glucose from carbs, it changes its metabolic state to depend on these ketones. The hallmark of ketosis is a shift in energy metabolism that can happen during times of fasting, vigorous activity, or—in the case of the zero-carb diet—by purposefully limiting the amount of carbohydrates consumed.

ADVANTAGES OF KETOSIS

Proponents of ketosis and the zero-carb diet point to several possible advantages. The main benefit is weight loss since the body uses its fat reserves as fuel. Furthermore, ketosis is thought to improve focus and mental clarity, which may improve cognitive function. Additionally, some people report having more energy and having better blood sugar control. People with some inflammatory illnesses may have better conditions as a result of the anti-inflammatory effects of ketosis.

TRACKING THE LEVELS OF KETONES

A critical component of any zero-carb diet is keeping an eye on your ketone levels if you want to get into and stay out of ketosis. Tests for ketones can be performed on breath, blood, or urine, among other materials. While urine strips are a popular and easily available method of monitoring ketosis, blood tests offer a more precise measurement of ketone levels. It's crucial to remember that different people will respond differently to a zero-carb diet and ketosis to varying degrees.

THE NECESSARY NUTRIENTS

Although the goal of a zero-carb diet is to cut out all carbohydrates, nutritional needs must also be met to avoid any possible deficits. Sustaining many body functions and preserving muscle mass depends on consuming an adequate amount of protein. When there are no carbs available, healthy fats like those found in avocados, almonds, and olive oil take over as the main energy source. Vegetables high in nutrients can still be added to supply vital vitamins, minerals, and fiber.

CRUCIAL ELEMENTS

Ensuring adequate consumption of vital nutrients is crucial, even while following a ketogenic or zero-carb diet. Minerals and vitamins like potassium, magnesium, and salt are essential for preserving the balance of electrolytes in the body and general health. It's also critical to drink enough water, particularly since ketosis can cause a rise in water loss.

POSSIBLE SHORTCOMINGS AND REMEDIES

Zero-carb diets have potential advantages, but if they are not properly monitored, they can result in inadequacies. Common problems include possible electrolyte imbalances and a fiber deficiency, which can affect intestinal health. These issues can be resolved by adding nutrient-rich foods like leafy greens and low-carb veggies or by supplementing. A well-rounded nutritional approach can be ensured and any inadequacies can be mitigated with regular monitoring of general health and consultation with healthcare professionals.

CHAPTER FOUR

APPLYING THE LOW-CARBOHYDRATE DIET

Carnivorous or all-meat diets, sometimes referred to as zero-carb diets, place a strong emphasis on avoiding carbs and substituting foods that are derived from animals. Although some animal products do include tiny amounts of carbohydrates, the phrase "zero carb" may not be entirely accurate, the main idea is to reduce carb intake as much as possible.

CARB-FREE FOODS

Foods with minimal or no carbohydrate content form the basis of the zero-carb diet. Foods that are approved usually consist of different types of meats, fish, poultry, and animal fats. For individuals on a zero-carb diet, core options include beef, hog, lamb, and fowl. Seafood can also be incorporated since fish and shellfish are often low in carbs. Because of their high carbohydrate content, dairy products are frequently avoided or restricted, while some people may have selected high-fat, low-carb dairy products.

AUTHORIZED MEATS

The mainstay of the zero-carb diet is meat. A range of cuts from beef, hog, lamb, and poultry are included in this. Processed meats, such as sausages and bacon, are also frequently used, but it's important to be aware of any preservatives or additions that could lead to hidden carbohydrates. Some followers of the ketogenic diet decide to use nutrient-dense organ meats like liver and kidney to get extra vitamins and minerals.

OILS AND FATS

Being a dense source of energy, fats are important in a zero-carb diet. Animal fats like tallow and lard as well as oils like olive and coconut oil are acceptable fats and oils. Low-carbohydrate options like butter and ghee are frequently utilized to boost the taste and richness of food. For people following a zero-carb diet, it is essential to maintain a sufficient intake of healthy fats because they support different physiological functions and assist in meeting energy requirements.

COCKTAILS

When following a zero-carb diet, water is usually the preferred beverage because it is both necessary for hydration and has no carbohydrates. Some people might also include unsweetened black coffee or tea, free of high-carbohydrate ingredients. When it comes to some diet sodas and artificial sweeteners, you should exercise caution since they can contain unidentified carbs that interfere with ketosis, a state in which the body burns fat for energy.

PLANNING MEALS

Meal planning for zero carbs entails choosing a range of animal-based foods and avoiding or eliminating products that contain carbohydrates. Organizing meals to feature a variety of meat, fish, and poultry cuts guarantees a varied intake of nutrients. Some people may decide to include time-restricted eating or intermittent fasting in their meal plans to improve the body's ability to enter and stay in a state of ketosis.

MAKING WELL-COMPOSED LOW-CARB MEALS

Ensuring a sufficient dose of fats and proteins is crucial to maintaining nutritional balance on a zero-carb diet. This balance can be attained by including a range of meats and sources of good fats. Despite the diet's naturally low carbohydrate content, it's important to pay attention to nutrient density and take supplements if the few food options don't provide enough of a certain vitamin or mineral. Maintaining a balanced, low-carb diet over time requires regular health monitoring and advice from a nutritionist or healthcare provider.

A zero-carb diet requires completely giving up all carbohydrates, including those found in fruits, vegetables, and grains. This is a drastic deviation from standard dietary guidelines. A sustainable meal plan that adheres to the zero-carb diet's tenets necessitates careful consideration of substitute nutrient sources.

EXAMPLES OF MENUS

Meat, seafood, eggs, and some dairy products are the mainstays of most zero-carb meal plans. Steak, poultry, or fish cooked in animal fats could be the main course of a sample supper, with possible side dishes including eggs and cheese.

Including organ meats can also supply important nutrients that a diet low in carbohydrates may be deficient in. To guarantee an adequate amount of energy, it is important to watch how much protein you eat and to select fatty cuts of meat.

SNACK SELECTION

With minimal carbs, it can be difficult to snack because typical snacks like fruits and crackers are off-limits. Given their high carbohydrate content, nuts—a popular snack in many diets—should normally be consumed in moderation. Rather, animal-based foods like cheese, hard-boiled eggs, and beef jerky are popular low-carb options. These snacks are a good supply of healthy fats and protein while still adhering to dietary limitations.

ON THE ZERO CARB DIET, DINING OUT

Making smart choices when dining out while following a zero-carb diet is necessary. The secret is to choose eateries that let you customize your meals and have a wide selection of meat-based dishes. Meats that have been roasted or grilled without additional sauces or coatings are usually safe options. To guarantee adherence to the zero-carb recommendations, it is crucial to express dietary preferences to the server clearly and concisely and to ask about ingredient lists and cooking methods.

GETTING AROUND RESTAURANTS

It's important to concentrate on unprocessed, whole foods when perusing restaurant menus and following a zero-carb diet. Restaurants that specialize in seafood, steakhouses, and a wide selection of meat options are frequently more flexible. It is crucial to stay away from starchy sides and sweet sauces; instead, choosing straightforward preparations like sautéed or grilled foods can support the diet's zero-carb purity. There might not be many options for salads, and as many dressings include added sugar, care should be taken while choosing one.

SOCIAL OCCASIONS AND LOW CARBOHYDRATES

Planning and communication may be necessary while following a zero-carb diet and participating in social events. Disclosing dietary restrictions to loved ones might help control expectations and prevent problems. When entertaining, bringing low-carb food items can help guarantee that there are appropriate selections. It's critical to create a balance between following the diet and socializing, making plans for events enjoyable without sacrificing dietary objectives.

Maintaining adaptability and being willing to make changes when needed will help make living a zero-carb lifestyle more pleasurable and sustainable.

CHAPTER FIVE

LOW CARB AND WELL-BEING

LOSING WEIGHT AND MANAGING IT

Many people have the desire to reach and maintain a healthy weight, which leads them to investigate different dietary strategies. One such strategy that is gaining popularity is the idea of extremely low-carb or zero-carb diets. These diets emphasize reducing or cutting out carbs in favor of consuming more fats and proteins as sources of energy. The basic premise is that the body enters a state of ketosis—where it burns fat stores for energy—when carbs are eliminated.

LOSING WEIGHT AND CUTTING CARBS

The idea behind the zero-carb weight loss strategy is to lower the body's insulin levels. The hormone insulin, which encourages the storage of fat, is released in response to the presence of carbohydrates, especially refined sugars. Proponents contend that cutting back on or eliminating carbohydrates keeps insulin levels low, urging the body to burn off its stored fat for energy. A zero-carb diet may cause some people to lose weight initially, but long-term success depends on things like consistent adherence, nutritional balance, and general lifestyle decisions.

SUSTAINING A PROPER WEIGHT

Eating the right kinds of food in moderation is just as important as eating a sufficient amount of it. Proponents of diets low in carbohydrates stress the value of emphasizing nutrient-dense foods including meat, fish, eggs, and some dairy products. Essential vitamins, minerals, and amino acids that promote general health can be found in these foods. However, it's important to proceed cautiously when it comes to eating zero carbs since it might make it difficult to meet dietary fiber requirements and get a variety of nutrients from plant sources.

PHYSICAL CAPABILITIES

The effect of a zero-carb diet on athletic performance is still up for discussion. Since high-intensity exercises primarily need the use of carbohydrates as fuel, some athletes contend that cutting out carbohydrates entirely could impair performance. Conversely, proponents of zero-carb diets contend that as the body adjusts to this nutritional strategy, it becomes more adept at using fats for energy. Since everyone reacts differently, it's critical for people who regularly exercise to keep an eye on their progress and modify their strategy as necessary.

ZERO CARB AND EXERCISE

A zero-carb lifestyle necessitates careful consideration of energy sources while incorporating exercise. While low-intensity activities can train the body to burn fat for fuel, high-intensity workouts might require a different strategy. Some people on a zero-carb diet time their carbohydrate intake strategically to fuel their workouts and achieve peak performance. A customized strategy that emphasizes adaptability and responsiveness to individual needs is needed to strike a balance between the demands of physical activity and the restrictions of a zero-carb diet.

There are several facets to the relationship between zero-carb diets and weight control, as well as how they affect athletic performance. These strategies may work for some people, but it's important to approach them mindful of your own needs, any potential nutritional gaps, and how sustainable these dietary choices may be in the long run. It is advisable to get advice from healthcare specialists and nutrition experts before making any significant lifestyle changes to ensure a well-rounded and health-conscious approach.

CHAPTER SIX

ATHLETES FOLLOWING A LOW-CARB DIET

A zero-carb diet is frequently adopted by athletes to improve both their general health and performance. It's imperative to carefully weigh the possible health effects of such a nutritional strategy, though.

CONSIDERATIONS FOR HEALTH

It's important to understand that not all athletes will benefit from a zero-carb diet, even though for some people it may result in quick weight loss and improved metabolic markers. The body uses carbohydrates as its main energy source, particularly while engaging in high-intensity activity. An athlete's capacity to maintain top performance may be impacted if the body is deprived of this essential fuel source.

BLOOD SUGAR CONTROL

The possible influence of a zero-carb diet on blood sugar management is one of the main causes of concern. Stable blood sugar levels depend on a constant supply of glucose, which is largely provided by carbohydrates. Athletes who consume insufficient amounts of carbohydrates may suffer from blood sugar swings, which can impair their overall athletic performance and cause weariness and lightheadedness.

EFFECT ON LEVELS OF CHOLESTEROL

Health experts disagree over the connection between cholesterol levels and a zero-carb diet. While some research indicates that cutting back on carbohydrates may enhance cholesterol profiles by raising HDL cholesterol, other studies contend that the lack of dietary fiber in carbohydrates may have negative consequences on cardiovascular health. To achieve a balanced approach to nutrition, athletes should closely monitor their cholesterol levels and seek advice from healthcare professionals.

POSSIBLE HAZARDS AND SAFETY MEASURES

A zero-carb diet may carry dangers, like insufficient fiber intake and nutritional deficits. In addition to providing energy, carbohydrates also add important vitamins, minerals, and dietary fiber to the diet. Deficits resulting from a lack of certain nutrients may have negative health implications. When adopting a zero-carb strategy, athletes should choose foods that are high in nutrients and, if needed, think about taking supplements to meet their nutritional requirements.

Moreover, before starting a zero-carb diet, athletes should speak with medical specialists, dietitians, or nutritionists. Individual differences in metabolic response and health status need to be considered. Tailored counsel can assist in reducing potential dangers and guarantee that dietary requirements are sufficiently satisfied.

Even though certain athletes may benefit from a zero-carb diet, it is important to approach this eating plan cautiously and be aware of any potential health risks.

CHAPTER SEVEN

PROLONGED DURABILITY

GETTING USED TO A LOW-CARB LIFESTYLE

The adoption of a zero-carb lifestyle necessitates a dramatic change in eating patterns and perspective. This strategy, which is based on cutting off carbohydrates from one's diet, calls for people to reconsider and reframe their relationship with food. Adopting a zero-carb lifestyle frequently means reducing or giving up typical carbohydrate sources like grains, fruits, and starchy vegetables in favor of foods high in protein and fat. This shift can be difficult since it requires departing from cultural customs and accepted dietary guidelines, which frequently call for a combination of macronutrients.

OVERCOMING OBSTACLES

Managing the physical and psychological components of a zero-carb lifestyle is necessary to overcome its hurdles. From a physiological standpoint, people could feel uncomfortable at first as their bodies become used to using fats and proteins rather than carbs as an energy source. Known as the "keto flu," this transition phase can cause headaches, irritability, and exhaustion. To overcome these obstacles, people must drink plenty of water, make sure they are getting enough electrolytes, and gradually transition to a low-carb lifestyle so that their bodies can adjust more easily.

Navigating social situations, where food choices frequently play a prominent role, is psychologically challenging. People who follow a zero-carb lifestyle may encounter mistrust or misunderstandings; therefore it's important for them to adequately convey their decisions. Creating a network of support and getting advice from specialists or others who share your values can help you adapt more successfully. Furthermore, focusing on the long-term advantages of increased energy, mental clarity, and general well-being can be a strong incentive to overcome the difficulties of a low-carb lifestyle.

CHOOSING TO EAT NO CARBS IN A SUSTAINABLE WAY

To make going zero-carb sustainable, one must take into account not only one's own health but also the larger effects on the environment and society. Although many people are motivated by the health benefits of a zero-carb lifestyle, sustainability is more than just good health. A more comprehensive approach to sustainability involves supporting local and sustainable farming practices, consuming food mindfully to minimize food waste, and sourcing animal products ethically.

Moreover, it is impossible to ignore how food decisions affect the ecosystem. Proponents of the low-carb lifestyle frequently highlight how animal agriculture may have a lower carbon footprint than some plant-based agricultural methods. But it's important to tackle this issue nuanced, taking into account things like land use, ecological impact overall, and regenerative farming methods. A sustainable zero-carb lifestyle requires striking a balance between environmental consciousness and personal health objectives.

Adopting a zero-carb lifestyle necessitates a significant change in eating patterns and the surmounting of psychological and physiological obstacles. Going zero-carb is a sustainable decision that takes into account not just one's health but also the environment, society, and ethics. Through the consideration of these factors, people can develop a zero-carb lifestyle that is sustainable, advantageous to their health, and supportive of sustainability as a whole.

CHAPTER EIGHT

OFTEN HELD MISCONCEPTIONS AND MYTHS

Many myths and misconceptions surround long-term sustainability, making it difficult to fully comprehend all of its complexities. The idea that adopting sustainable practices means forgoing economic growth is one common misconception. Sustainability is a well-rounded strategy that takes into account social, economic, and environmental aspects. It is important to promote inclusive and resilient development rather than stalling progress.

Another widespread misunderstanding that contributes to people's sense of helplessness is the idea that individual acts have little bearing on sustainability. This is untrue; individual decisions have a collective impact on important environmental and social consequences. Over time, small behavioral adjustments like cutting back on energy use or choosing environmentally friendly products can add up to a big impact.

Another common misconception is the idea that sustainability issues can only be resolved by technological innovation. Although technology is important, a complete strategy calls for systemic and societal changes. Relying solely on technological advancements may lead to overlooking behavioral and structural aspects that are equally crucial for achieving long-term sustainability.

ADDRESSING CRITICISMS

Criticism towards long-term sustainability initiatives often centers around their perceived impracticality and economic burden. Some argue that prioritizing sustainability may compromise economic growth, particularly in industries traditionally dependent on resource-intensive practices. However, evidence suggests that sustainable practices can enhance efficiency

Innovation driven by sustainability goals can lead to cost savings and new business opportunities.

Another criticism is that global cooperation for sustainability is unrealistic due to geopolitical tensions and conflicting interests. While achieving universal consensus is undoubtedly challenging, there is a growing recognition that interconnected global challenges require collaborative solutions. Regional and international agreements, as well as grassroots movements, demonstrate the potential for collective action to address sustainability issues.

The criticism of green washing, where companies present a misleading image of their environmental efforts, is also pertinent. To address this, transparency and accountability are crucial. Stricter regulations, certification systems, and consumer awareness can contribute to holding entities accountable for genuinely sustainable practices.

CLARIFYING MISINFORMATION

Misinformation about sustainability often arises from oversimplified narratives or incomplete information. One common area of confusion is the belief that sustainable practices are prohibitively expensive.

While there may be initial costs, many sustainable initiatives result in long-term economic benefits. Investing in renewable energy, for example, can lead to substantial savings on energy costs over time.

Another area of misinformation revolves around the idea that sustainability is a one-size-fits-all concept. In reality, contextual factors, such as geographical location, cultural considerations, and resource availability, play a crucial role in determining the most effective sustainability strategies. Tailoring approaches to specific contexts ensures that solutions are realistic and adaptable.

There is also a prevalent misconception that sustainability is solely an environmental concern. In truth, sustainability encompasses social and economic dimensions. A holistic approach considers the well-being of communities, social equity, and economic resilience alongside environmental conservation.

Dispelling common myths, addressing criticisms, and clarifying misinformation are essential steps toward fostering a more nuanced and accurate understanding of long-term sustainability. Embracing a comprehensive perspective that integrates environmental, social, and economic considerations is key to building a sustainable future.

CHAPTER NINE

MEAL IDEAS AND RECIPES

ZERO CARB BREAKFASTS

For individuals adhering to a low-carb or ketogenic lifestyle, crafting a breakfast that is entirely devoid of carbs might seem like a challenge, but it's entirely possible. Eggs, being a versatile and nutritious option, take center stage in zero-carb breakfasts. Whether scrambled, fried, or poached, eggs provide a solid protein foundation with zero carbs. Incorporating high-fat options such as bacon or sausage can elevate the meal's flavor profile while remaining carb-free. Additionally, incorporating ingredients like avocado, cheese, and smoked salmon can add healthy fats and variety to the meal without introducing carbs.

PROTEIN-PACKED OPTIONS

A protein-packed breakfast is essential for sustained energy throughout the day. Including a variety of protein sources ensures a well-rounded meal that not only satisfies hunger but also supports muscle health. Options such as Greek yogurt, cottage cheese, and protein-rich smoothies can be excellent choices. Eggs, whether in omelets, frittatas, or boiled, are a classic protein source that can be paired with vegetables to enhance nutritional content. For those seeking a plant-based protein boost, incorporating nuts, seeds, and tofu can be both satisfying and nutritious.

ENERGIZING SMOOTHIES

Smoothies offer a convenient and delicious way to kickstart the day with a burst of energy. To keep them low in carbs, opt for unsweetened almond or coconut milk as a base. Adding high-protein ingredients like protein powder, Greek yogurt, or nut butter contributes to a more filling and energizing beverage. Include low-carb fruits such as berries or avocado for flavor and additional nutrients. To enhance the texture and nutritional content, consider incorporating leafy greens like spinach or kale.

This not only adds a vibrant color but also provides essential vitamins and minerals.

ZERO CARB LUNCHES AND DINNERS

Crafting satisfying and flavorful lunches and dinners without carbs requires a focus on protein and healthy fats. Grilled and roasted meats, such as chicken, beef, or pork, take center stage, offering a delicious and filling main course. Fish, particularly fatty fish like salmon or mackerel, not only provides a protein boost but also delivers omega-3 fatty acids. Accompanying these main dishes with non-starchy vegetables like broccoli, cauliflower, or asparagus adds fiber, vitamins, and minerals without significantly contributing to carb intake.

GRILLED AND ROASTED MEATS

Grilling and roasting meats are cooking techniques that not only enhance flavors but also contribute to a satisfying and low-carb meal. Meats like steak, chicken, and pork can be marinated with herbs, spices, and olive oil to add depth and richness without increasing carb content. Grilling vegetables alongside the meats imparts a smoky flavor and provides a complementary side dish. The charring from grilling and the caramelization from roasting contribute to a visually appealing and flavorful dining experience.

SATISFYING SIDE DISHES

Sides play a crucial role in rounding out a low-carb meal, providing additional nutrients and textures. Non-starchy vegetables, both raw and cooked, serve as excellent side dish options. Roasted Brussels sprouts with bacon or sautéed spinach with garlic are flavorful choices that complement the main protein source. Cauliflower, being a versatile vegetable, can be transformed into mashed cauliflower or cauliflower rice, mimicking traditional carb-heavy sides without sacrificing taste.

www.ingramcontent.com/pod-product-compliance
Lightning Source LLC
Chambersburg PA
CBHW050748260726
48661CB00001B/477